COPING WITH PREGNANCY LOSS

A Guide to Healing After Miscarriage and Stillbirth

James Edwards

TABLE OF CONTENTS

INTRODUCTION

There is an intense and often silent pain in the quiet corners of our hearts, one that words cannot explain and people who have never experienced it will find it difficult to understand. It is the intense pain of miscarriage and stillbirth. This pain affects the lives of countless individuals and couples, leaving a complex variety of emotions, questions, and aching emptiness as a result. We often find ourselves roving through the shadowed valleys of grief as we commence on the journey to healing after such a painful loss, searching for the subtle path toward renewal and hope.

'COPING WITH PREGNANCY LOSS: A GUIDE TO HEALING AFTER MISCARRIAGE AND STILLBIRTH' is a book dedicated to those who have suffered the heartbreak of miscarriage or stillbirth. It is a beacon of hope in the darkest of times, a companion on the road to recovery, and a haven of compassion for those seeking comfort and understanding. We delve into the depths of grief here, addressing the wide range of emotions that come with loss, from sadness and anger to guilt and confusion. We recognize the unique, personal nature of each person's journey and offer unconditional support, understanding that healing is not a linear process and that each step forward is a victory.

The way to recovery after miscarriage or stillbirth is a difficult one, but it is also one that can lead to newfound strength, resiliency, and joy. By gently reminding you that the human spirit has an amazing capacity to heal, flourish, and find comfort even in the wake of intense sorrow, 'COPING WITH PREGNANCY LOSS' invites you to travel this way. This book is proof that the human heart can once more blossom with love, resiliency, and hope even in the face of life's most heartbreaking moments.

CHAPTER ONE

Basic Knowledge of Pregnancy Loss

Pregnancy loss is a sad and often baffling experience. It can be difficult to understand the plenty of disturbing emotions and questions that follow. In this chapter, we will look at pregnancy loss in all of its forms, including miscarriage and stillbirth, in the hopes of shedding light on the tough journey of healing that follows.

Range of Pregnancy Loss

Pregnancy loss includes a broad range of experiences, from early miscarriages to late-term stillbirths. Each loss is specific and deeply personal, and it is important to understand that there is no one-size-fits-all approach to coping with the agonizing pain that comes with it. Let's look at the various types of pregnancy loss:

1. Miscarriage:

A miscarriage occurs when a pregnancy is lost before the fifth month. It can happen for a variety of reasons, the most common of which are genetic abnormalities, hormonal imbalances, or other medical conditions. The majority of miscarriages occur during the first trimester, often before a woman begins to feel the weight and joy of pregnancy. A miscarriage has a remarkable emotional impact, even if it occurs early in pregnancy.

2. Stillbirth:

A stillbirth occurs when a pregnancy is lost after the fifth month, usually during the second or third trimester. Stillbirth can be caused by different conditions, including placental problems, infections, and other medical complications. Stillbirth is a sad event because it frequently occurs after parents have formed a firm emotional bond with their unborn child.

Coping with the Loss of a Pregnancy

Understanding the nature of pregnancy loss is important, but so is investigating how individuals and couples can cope with their sorrow. Grieving a pregnancy loss is a specific and highly personal experience, but there is a common cord that binds those who have gone through it.

Emotions and Grief

Grief is a natural reaction to the loss of a pregnancy. It is important to understand that there is no 'right' way to grieve and that everyone's journey is specific to himself or herself. Among the most common emotions experienced during pregnancy loss are:

(a) Sadness: It is natural to feel an intense sense of loss and sadness. Allowing yourself to feel these emotions without judgment is important.

(b) Guilt: Many people feel guilty and wonder if they could have done something different to avoid the pregnancy loss. It's important for you to keep in mind that pregnancy loss is almost never the result of anything you did or did not do.

(c) Anger: You can be angry at yourself, your partner, or even the universe. It is acceptable to feel this emotion, but the important thing is to express it in a healthy manner.

(d) Isolation: It's natural to feel isolated as if no one understands your pain. However, it's important for you to reach out to supportive friends, family, or support groups for assistance.

(e) Anxiety and Fear: The fear and the worry in relation to losing future pregnancies can be devastating. It's important for you to seek professional help or join a support group that can help you manage these emotions.

Expressing Your Anger

Because each person involved may experience grief differently, pregnancy loss can have an obvious impact on relationships. It's important to communicate clearly with your partner and loved ones. Express your emotions, listen to their stories, and remember that everyone copes differently.

Seeking Professional Assistance

When going through the disturbing agony of pregnancy loss, therapists, counselors, and support groups can be invaluable resources. They offer a safe place to express your feelings as well as advice on coping and healing.

Finally, understanding pregnancy loss is the first step in the healing process. Whether you've had a miscarriage or a stillbirth, the emotions you're experiencing are understandable, and you're not alone in your grief. In the following chapters, we will look at various ways to heal and find solace after a pregnancy loss, as well as ways to remember and honor the children who were taken too soon. Remember that even in the darkest of times, healing is possible and hope can be found.

CHAPTER TWO

The Healing Journey

Healing after a pregnancy loss, whether a miscarriage or stillbirth, is a deeply personal and often difficult way to travel. It is a path marked by grief, pain, and resilience, but it can also lead to a thorough transformation and growth. In this chapter, we will look at various aspects of the healing process, offering advice, support, and hope to those who have suffered the agonizing pain of a pregnancy loss.

Recognizing the Pain

Recognizing the pain is the first step in the healing process. Pregnancy loss can feel like an emotional earthquake that shakes the foundation of your world. It is important to recognize that your grief is valid and that there is no right or wrong way to feel. Your feelings could range from deep sadness and anger to guilt, confusion, and even numbness. It's important for you to embrace this feeling without much reasoning.

It's important to be aware that healing does not imply forgetting. It's okay to carry your loss with you as you move forward because it's a part of your story. Recognizing the pain is the first step toward resolving it.

Obtaining Assistance

You are not alone on this journey. Seek the help of friends, family, or a therapist who specializes in pregnancy loss. It can be extremely healing to share your feelings and experiences with others who have been through similar situations. Online and in-person support groups can provide a sense of community and understanding that you may not find elsewhere.

If you have a partner, they are also dealing with grief. During this difficult time, open and honest communication can help you both process your emotions and strengthen your bond.

Self-Compassion

Self-compassion is essential during the healing process. Be gentle with yourself and recognize that healing is not a straight line. There will be good and bad days, which is completely normal. Take the time to look after your physical and emotional health. Relaxation exercises, journaling, engaging in activities that bring you joy, or simply allowing yourself to rest when you need it are all examples of this.

Memorials and Rituals

Creating rituals or memorials to honor your lost pregnancy and unborn child can be a healing process. Lighting a candle, planting a tree, or keeping a journal can help you come to terms with your loss and remember your baby in a meaningful way. These rituals can also serve as a source of encouragement and relief in painful times.

Looking for Meaning and Purpose

As you progress through your healing process, you may begin to seek meaning and purpose in your experiences. Finding meaning can be a deeply personal process. Some people may engage in the work of assisting to raise awareness about pregnancy loss or donate to organizations that assist others facing similar difficulties. Others may find meaning in their own personal development, learning, or creative endeavors as a result of their grief.

The Path to Hope

Though the path to healing after a pregnancy loss is marked by pain and loss, it also has the potential for hope and renewal. The pain may become more bearable with time, and the healing process may result in a renewed sense of purpose and appreciation for life.

Remember that each person's healing is unique. There is no set timeline, and it is normal to experience a range of emotions as you chart your own course. You have more strength, resilience, and healing capacity than you realize.

Hold onto the belief that there is light at the end of the tunnel, and that with time, you will find your way back to a place of peace, love, and hope.

CHAPTER THREE

Coping with Loss

Grief is a complex and deeply personal emotion that is unique to each person and situation. When a pregnancy is lost, whether through miscarriage or stillbirth, the grief experienced is extremely complex. In this chapter, we will look at the many facets of grief and discuss coping strategies to help you maneuver this difficult path to healing.

Understanding Loss

Grief is not a straight line. It ebbs and flows, crashing like waves against your soul's shore. It is a natural reaction to loss and usually occurs in stages. These stages are defined by the well-known Kübler-Ross model as denial, anger, bargaining, depression, and acceptance. Grief, on the other hand, is rarely this neat and predictable. It's more like a web, with different emotions entwining and overlapping. It's perfectly normal to feel sad one moment and angry the next.

The grief you feel after a miscarriage is unique because it represents the loss of dreams, hopes, and the future you imagined for your child. It is important to acknowledge that your grief is valid and that there is no right or wrong way to grieve.

Coping Techniques

1. Allow Yourself to Grieve: Recognizing and accepting your feelings is the first step in coping with grief. Allow yourself to grieve without judgment. Grief is not a sign of weakness; it is proof of the love you had for your child that you never saw.

2. Seek Help: You don't have to go through this alone. Make contact with friends, family, or pregnancy loss support groups. Talking with others who have suffered a similar loss can be extremely reassuring.

3. Professional Assistance: Grief can be overwhelming at times, leading to mental health issues such as depression or intense worry. Do not be afraid to seek the advice of a grief and loss therapist or counselor.

4. Create Rituals: Many people find solace in creating rituals or memorial services to honor their lost child's memory. This can be a meaningful way to say goodbye and bring things to a close.

5. Express Your Feelings: Find ways to express your feelings, whether through journaling, art, or other creative outlets. Writing letters to your child, making a scrapbook, or painting can all be therapeutic and healing activities.

6. Self-Care: Look after your physical and emotional health. Rest, nutrition, and exercise should be prioritized. Grief can be physically draining, and taking care of yourself can help you regain some of your strength.

7. Have Realistic Expectations: Recognize that healing takes time. Be gentle with yourself and accept that you may never truly overcome the loss, but you can learn to live with it and find joy in your life again.

8. Concentrate on the Positive: While it may appear difficult, try to concentrate on the positive aspects of your life. Celebrate your love for your child, no matter how short their time with you was.

9. Plan for the Future: You may decide to try for another pregnancy in the future. Consult with your healthcare provider to develop a plan that is appropriate for both you and your partner. Remember that this is a deeply personal decision with no right or wrong answer.

10. Honor Your Child's Memory: Find ways to keep your child's memory alive in your heart. You could make a donation in their honor to a charity, plant a tree, or participate in pregnancy loss awareness events.

In conclusion, dealing with grief after a pregnancy loss is a journey that requires patience, self-compassion, and support. Remember that healing is about learning to carry the weight of your loss while still moving forward, not forgetting. Grief has no timetable, and your experience is unique to you. You will eventually find a way to honor your child's memory while also rediscovering hope and happiness.

CHAPTER FOUR

Types and Causes of Pregnancy Loss

The devastating experience of losing a pregnancy affects countless people and families all over the world. It includes a variety of situations and states, each with its own specific causes and psychological ramifications. One of the most important steps in the healing process following a miscarriage, stillbirth, or any other type of pregnancy loss is realizing the various kinds and causes of pregnancy loss. In order to assist individuals and couples in maneuvering their journey of grief and recovery, this chapter explores these categories and sheds light on the factors that contribute to pregnancy loss.

Types of Pregnancy Loss

1. Miscarriage: Within the first five months of pregnancy, miscarriage is the most common type of pregnancy loss. It frequently involves the death of an embryo or fetus before it has a chance to grow into a healthy child. There are various categories into which miscarriages can be divided, such as:

(a) Chemical pregnancy: This type of pregnancy develops soon after conception and ends before an ultrasound can confirm it. It frequently results in a slightly heavier or delayed menstrual cycle.

(b) Blighted Ovum: An implanted fertilized egg that fails to develop into an embryo in the uterus.

(c) Threatened Miscarriage: In situations where cramps and/or bleeding are present but the pregnancy may still be viable.

(d) Undoubtedly Unavoidable Miscarriage: When there is absolute certainty that the pregnancy will end.

2. Stillbirth: A pregnancy that ends after five months of gestation is referred to as a stillbirth. Complex causes such as genetic, placental, or fetal abnormalities can result in stillbirth.

3. Ectopic Pregnancy: When a fertilized egg implants outside of the uterus, usually in the fallopian tube, the result is an ectopic pregnancy. This illness is incurable and needs to be treated right away to avoid potentially fatal complications.

4. Molar Pregnancy: This uncommon ailment is characterized by the formation of an irregular mass of tissue in place of a viable embryo. Medical intervention is required to stop the growth of cancerous cells.

5. Recurrent Pregnancy Loss: Multiple pregnancy losses are categorized as recurrent pregnancy loss and can occur in certain individuals. Numerous factors, such as genetic, hormonal, or anatomical problems, could be the cause of this.

Reasons for Losing Pregnancy

Determining the reasons behind pregnancy loss is a difficult and frequently emotionally taxing process. Even though it's normal to look for solutions, it's highly essential to understand that sometimes the source is still unknown. Pregnancy loss may be caused by the following:

1. Chromosomal Abnormalities: When an embryo or fetus has an abnormally high or low number of chromosomes, it is the most common cause of miscarriage. These anomalies are uncontrollable and frequently happen at random.

2. Maternal Health Conditions: Pregnancy loss can be exacerbated by conditions like diabetes, autoimmune diseases, thyroid issues, and polycystic ovary syndrome (PCOS).

3. Infections: Some infections, such as those that are transmitted sexually, can cause pregnancy loss. Maintaining appropriate prenatal care is essential to preventing and treating such problems.

4. Uterine Abnormalities: It may be difficult for a pregnancy to start or continue if there are abnormalities in the uterine structure.

5. Hormonal Imbalances: The uterus's capacity to sustain a pregnancy may be impacted by hormonal imbalances, particularly those involving progesterone.

6. Environmental Factors: Pregnancy loss may be more likely in people who are exposed to toxins, radiation, or specific medications.

7. Lifestyle Decisions: Pregnancy loss can be caused by smoking, drinking alcohol, using drugs, and consuming too much caffeine.

8. Advanced Maternal Age: Age-related factors put women over 35 at higher risk of miscarrying a child.

9. Psychological Stress: Although it is not a direct cause, long-term stress negatively impacts general health and well-being, which in turn can influence pregnancy outcomes.

For some people, knowing the precise reason behind a pregnancy loss can terminate their agony, but for others, it might not make sense. Healing is a journey that requires accepting the uncertainty of pregnancy loss and finding comfort in the help of family, friends, and medical professionals.

CHAPTER FIVE

Repeated Loss of Pregnancy

Nobody plans to go on the journey known as recurrent pregnancy loss (RPL). It's a storm that keeps threatening to submerge your dreams and aspirations. I want you to know that you are not alone as you read this chapter in our book about healing after miscarriage and stillbirth. Recurrent pregnancy loss presents difficulties for many people, including couples. It's important to understand that by sharing our stories with other people who are undergoing the same problem, we can draw strength and comfort from one another.

Understanding Repeated Pregnancy Loss

The occurrence of three or more consecutive miscarriages before the fifth month of gestation is referred to as recurrent pregnancy loss. It is a devastating emotional experience, frequently accompanied by feelings of despair, confusion, and frustration. RPL can be a daunting experience, but it is important to remember that healing and hope are possible.

Emotional Highs and Lows During Recurrent Pregnancy Loss

Dealing with recurrent pregnancy loss can have a negative impact on your emotional well-being. You may feel a variety of emotions, ranging from sadness and anger to guilt and confusion. These feelings are completely normal, and acknowledging them is the first step toward recovery. It is important to find a safe space where you can express your emotions and fears without fear of being judged. This could be with a supportive partner, a friend, or a pregnancy loss therapist.

Looking for Solutions

A common reaction to recurrent pregnancy loss is the search for answers. You might want to investigate the cause and come up with a solution. It is critical to seek the advice of a healthcare provider who specializes in reproductive medicine. They will run a battery of tests to rule out any potential causes of your miscarriages, such as hormonal imbalances, genetic abnormalities, uterine issues, or immune system issues.

Remember that it is not your fault during this diagnostic phase. These losses were not caused by you. Be kind to yourself and open to exploring potential treatment options.

Treatment and Assistance

Depending on the underlying causes, various treatment options may be available. These treatments could include hormonal therapies, surgery, or lifestyle changes. It is important to consult with your healthcare provider to determine the best course of action for your particular situation.

Lean on your support system throughout this process, and consider joining a support group for people who have experienced recurrent pregnancy loss. Connecting with others who have been through similar experiences can provide invaluable insight, understanding, and encouragement.

Accepting Self-Care

The experience of recurrent pregnancy loss can be tiresome. As you go through medical appointments, treatments, and emotional turbulence, it's easy to lose sight of your own well-being. Make self-care a top priority during this trying time. Yoga, meditation, journaling, and seeking comfort in nature are examples of such activities. Remember that self-care is a necessary act of self-preservation, not selfishness.

Taking the Next Step

Repeated pregnancy loss may delay your journey to parenthood. It may inspire you to pursue alternative methods, such as adoption or surrogacy, or it may motivate you to advocate for RPL research and support. Accept that healing can take many forms and that your journey is unique to you.

In conclusion, recurrent pregnancy loss is a terrifying storm, but the clouds can part to reveal rays of hope with time, support, and perseverance. Remember that your story demonstrates your resilience and strength. This chapter in our book is dedicated to you, the survivors of recurrent pregnancy loss, and serves as a reminder that even the most difficult storms in life can be overcome.

CHAPTER SIX

Self-Treatment and Recovery Following Pregnancy Loss

Healing after any kind of pregnancy loss, like miscarriage and stillbirth, is frequently a difficult and intensely personal process. Feelings can be overpowering, and the physical toll can drain you. This chapter is devoted to the practice of self-healing and self-care, recognizing that these qualities are essential for maneuvering the road to recovery.

Practicing Self-Care

Self-care is a great aid in times of grief and healing, not just a fashionable term. Your path is distinct, and the way you choose to take care of yourself can have a remarkable impact on the healing process. In order to integrate self-care into your life at a time of pregnancy loss, you will need to observe the following key points:

1. Accept Your Emotions: Accept and embrace your emotions, whether they are sadness, anger, guilt, or a variety of other emotions. They are all valid and necessary parts of your healing process.

2. Seek Help: Rely on your support network, which could include friends, family, a therapist, or support groups. Sharing your feelings and experiences can be extremely therapeutic.

3. Rest and Recuperation: Allow your body the time it requires to physically heal. Rest and recuperation are essential, so don't be afraid to ask for assistance with daily tasks and responsibilities in order to have the necessary time to rest.

4. Nourish Your Body: Nutritious foods and adequate hydration are essential for physical recovery. Pay attention to your body's needs and feed it accordingly.

5. Engage in Mindful Exercise: Low-impact activities such as yoga or strolling can reduce both mental and physical stress. You can seek advice from your healthcare provider for exercises that are good for you.

6. Mindfulness and Meditation: Practicing mindfulness and meditation can help you maintain your composure and control your stress and anxiety.

7. Creativity and Art: You can express your feelings and find comfort through creative outlets like writing, painting, or music.

Accepting Healing

Healing is a continuous process rather than a final result. After losing a pregnancy, try these strategies for nurturing a sense of growth and healing:

1. Create Rituals: Establish private rituals that pay tribute to your deceased loved one and offer a sense of closure. A scrapbook dedication, a tree planting, or a candle lighting can all be heartfelt ways to honor your child.

2. Educate Yourself: You can enhance healing and demystify your experience by being aware of the emotional and physical components of pregnancy loss. There is

a need to speak with medical experts or support groups to get more details on the issue of pregnancy loss.

3. Journaling: You can better understand your thoughts and feelings by keeping a journal. Put your experiences, aspirations, worries, and dreams in writing. It can give you direction and make it easier to monitor your development.

4. Have patience with yourself: There will be ups and downs on the healing journey; it is not a straight line. At the tough times, remember to treat yourself with kindness and patience.

5. Find Meaning: Try to make sense of what happened to you. It may inspire you to advocate for an increased understanding of pregnancy loss, provide support for those who experience it, or give your life new meaning.

6. Appreciate Little Wins: Little wins can be had every day. Every accomplishment, whether it's getting out of bed, eating, or spending time with a friend, should be acknowledged.

Maintaining Close Relationships

Losing a pregnancy has an impact on the person experiencing it as well as those around them. Be open in your communication with your family, friends, and partner. It's important for you to recognize and appreciate the fact that they are also grieving as you are, and be mindful of how you approach them in communication.

(a) Support for Partners: Talk openly with your spouse, understanding that you may experience grief in different ways. Rely on one another for support, and if necessary, think about seeking professional counseling.

(b) Friends and Family: Tell the people you care about your needs and boundaries.
Tell them how they can assist you most, if it's just by lending a sympathetic ear,
offering a helping hand, or providing space when you need it.

(c) Support Groups: It can be very beneficial to join a support group for pregnancy
loss. There are people in the community that genuinely get what you're going
through.

Self-care and healing are essential components of the grieving process. Accept the
process, nourish your body and soul, and reach out to the people who can help you.
As you honor the memory of the child you lost and nurture hope for the future, you
will eventually find your own path to healing and resilience.

CHAPTER SEVEN

Attempting Once More

Healing after a pregnancy loss, whether miscarriage or stillbirth is a deeply personal and often agonizing journey. It's a journey that no one ever expects to take, but so many do. This chapter will look at the difficult and emotional decision to try again. It's a decision fraught with hope, fear, and uncertainty, but it's a critical step toward healing.

The Burden of Loss

Miscarriage or stillbirth can leave an indelible mark on your heart and soul. The heaviness of grief and the deprivation it leaves behind can be crushing. It's natural to wonder if you'll ever be able to bear the thought of experiencing such agony again. Many women who have been through this sad experience are debating whether to try for another pregnancy.

The pain of loss frequently lingers, and it is never completely forgotten or healed. What you thought would be an easy transition into parenthood is now an ordeal of emotions. "Is it worth trying again?" you may wonder. "Can I deal with the fear, uncertainty, and the possibility of experiencing loss again?"

The Influence of Hope

Despite the deep grief and emotional scars that a miscarriage can leave, there is something powerful about hope. Hope has a unique ability to heal and sustain us. Even in the darkest of times, it's the tiny flame that refuses to go out.

The character of hope can assist you in making the decision to try again. The desire to one day hold a healthy baby in your arms, to complete the family you've always wanted, or simply to enjoy the joy and wonder of pregnancy. This hope can be a powerful force that propels you forward, encouraging you to take the risk.

Confronting Fear

Trying again after a miscarriage takes enormous courage. It entails facing the fear that has likely plagued you since your loss. Fear of another loss, disappointment, or enduring the same heartache again. These concerns are entirely reasonable, and acknowledging them is an important part of the healing process.

It's important to remember that your fear is a reflection of your love for the child you lost. Your fear reminds you of the strong bond you formed during that pregnancy. By acknowledging and confronting your fear, you can begin to address it and possibly even lessen its hold on you.

Seeking Assistance

Remember that you don't have to make this decision alone as you consider trying again. Seek the assistance of a trusted friend or a therapist who specializes in pregnancy loss and grief. Openly discussing your feelings, fears, and hopes can be extremely therapeutic.

It is also important to have an open dialogue with your healthcare provider. They can inform you about your specific situation, potential risks, and ways to improve your odds of having a healthy pregnancy. As you commence on this new journey, your medical team can be an invaluable source of guidance and reassurance.

A Journey Designed Specifically for You

The decision to try again is deeply personal, and no one-size-fits-all solution exists. It's your journey, and it's perfectly fine to take your time making this decision. Whether you decide to try again right away or after months or even years, the decision should be made when you feel ready and when your hope outweighs your fear.

Ultimately, attempting again following the loss of a pregnancy is a sign of your courage, resiliency, and optimistic spirit. It's a step toward healing, one that recognizes the love you have for your kid who has passed away and the opportunities that still exist.

In conclusion, the choice to retry after a miscarriage is a significant and intensely personal one. This decision is a representation of love, hope, and the resiliency of the human spirit. Remind yourself that you are not alone on this journey as you consider your options. Seek assistance, rely on those you love, and have faith in your own abilities. The constant force of hope remains in the face of loss, fear, and uncertainty.

CHAPTER EIGHT

Respecting Your Infant's Memory

A stillbirth or miscarriage results in the loss of a child, which is an extremely painful and heartbreaking experience. Honoring your baby's presence in your life is a potent way to find comfort and preserve their memory as you travel the healing path. We'll look at a number of ways in this chapter to memorialize your beloved child and allow their memory to serve as a source of inspiration and comfort as you work toward healing.

1. Refer to and Name Your Child

No matter how short their life was, your baby existed and had significance. If you haven't already, giving them a name is one way to pay tribute to their memory.

Giving your child a name can help you feel at peace and acknowledge their special existence. By naming your child something meaningful to you, you can make their memory a physical part of your family.

2. Establish a Memorial Area

Creating a memorial area in your house can function as a sacred place where you can remember your child. You can dedicate an entire room, or just a corner of it, to your baby's memory. Decorate it with special objects that represent your child's presence in your life, such as photos, candles, artwork, or mementos. You can use this area as a place to grieve, reflect, and find a sense of connection to your child.

3. Establish an honorary garden

If you find comfort in nature, creating a memorial garden is a lovely way to honor your baby's memory. In honor of your child, plant flowers or trees in a designated area of your yard or a neighboring park. Watching the plants flourish and remembering your child's life can bring you comfort as they grow and bloom. A plaque or unique stone engraved with your baby's name and a heartfelt message can also be used to add personal touches to the garden.

4. Compose a Journal or Letter

Writing down your ideas and emotions can be a healing way to pay tribute to your child. Try expressing your love and sorrow in a letter to your child. To record your healing process and your aspirations for the future, you can also keep a journal. This can be a remembrance of your child and a way to honor their influence on your life for years to come.

5. Produce Art or Memorabilia

If you have artistic talent, think about making souvenirs or artwork that honors your child. You can create custom jewelry with your child's name or birthstone, or you can paint, draw, or sculpt something that symbolizes them. These artistic endeavors can serve as a therapeutic means of honoring your child and commemorating their existence.

6. Take Part in Altruistic Pursuits

Serving others in remembrance of their child brings comfort to many parents. Take into consideration participating in philanthropic endeavors pertaining to miscarriage and neonatal care. To help people going through similar experiences, you can volunteer your time, donate to organizations, or take part in fundraisers. When you volunteer your time positively influencing the lives of others, you will not only be paying tribute to your baby's memory but also assisting in finding meaning in your own loss.

7. Conduct a Memorial Service

You can celebrate and remember your baby's life with friends and family at a memorial ceremony. Readings, music, or rituals that are particularly meaningful to you and your loved ones can be added to make the occasion uniquely yours. It's an opportunity for you to communicate your emotions, share memories, and enlist the help of people who love you.

In conclusion, remembering your baby is a very healing and intimate journey. It enables you to come up with strategies for preserving your child's presence in your house and heart. Even though you may never fully recover from a loss, these tributes can offer you consolation, motivation, and inspiration while you move forward with your recovery. In addition to serving as a constant reminder of the love and bond you two had, your baby's memory can serve as evidence of the courage and resiliency you've gained via your journey through bereavement and recovery.

CHAPTER NINE

Considering the Future

Following a miscarriage or stillbirth, the future may seem vague and the way forward may be cloaked in a mixture of fear, hope, and grief. You have begun to lay the groundwork for healing as you have journeyed through the preceding chapters, delving into the profound depths of your pain. We will be concentrating on looking forward, reviving hope, and creating a new life that honors the suffering and the opportunities that lie ahead in this chapter.

Accepting Hope

Hope is a strong emotion. Even the deepest wounds can be healed by it. Hope can guide you toward healing even though your grief may still be a constant presence in your life. In order to embrace hope as you consider the future, consider the following:

1. Self-Compassion: A reminder to treat yourself with kindness. Grief has no set time frame, and healing takes time. Recognize your suffering, but also your courage and resiliency.

2. Creating Realistic Goals: Give yourself a list of modest, doable objectives. These could be as easy as getting out of bed in the morning, taking a quick stroll, or making new friends. With time, these tiny victories will boost your self-assurance.

3. Develop a Vision: Give your future some thought. How would you like it to appear? How would you like to feel? Which goals and desires do you still have? This activity can assist you in regaining a sense of direction.

4. Support System: Be in the company of people who are sympathetic to and understanding of your healing process. Having a support system, whether it be via friends, family, support groups, or therapy, is highly essential.

5. Seeking Professional Assistance: Don't be afraid to get assistance from a mental health professional if you're having trouble controlling your grief or your emotional state. Counseling can offer helpful direction and assistance.

Respecting Your Absent Child

The gloomy mood associated with miscarriage or stillbirth never fully goes away, but it can coexist with hope and happiness. Paying tribute to your deceased child is one way to find comfort on your journey ahead:

1. Memorialize: Construct a tribute or memento honoring your child's life. This could be something tangible, like jewelry or artwork, or it could be a symbolic act, like planting a tree or designating a room in your house for this purpose.

2. Tell Your Story: Telling others about your experiences can help many people find healing. For those who have suffered similar losses, your story can offer consolation and hope. Think about sharing your story in writing or speaking.

3. Acts of Kindness: One lovely way to preserve your child's spirit is to carry out acts of kindness in their honor. You could volunteer, make a charitable donation, or launch a project that honors your child's legacy.

Creating New Starts

You might find that your journey involves unanticipated blessings and fresh starts as you look to the future. Here are a few strategies for seizing these chances:

1. Rainbow Baby: A child born after a loss is referred to as a "rainbow baby" by those who want to try for another child. It represents optimism and the possibility of a fresh start.

2. Personal Growth: Make the most of this time by concentrating on your own learning and development. Investigate your interests, take up new hobbies, and learn new abilities. It's an opportunity to get back in touch with your dreams and self.

3. Advocacy and Support: Some people find meaning in pushing for increased understanding and support for bereaved mothers. In your community and beyond, you have the power to advocate for change.

4. Building Resilience: The suffering you've gone through has given you extraordinary strength. Make use of this resilience to move forward with renewed resolve in the future.

In conclusion, planning for the future following a stillbirth or miscarriage is a difficult and sensitive process. Every person's journey is different, molded by their dreams and experiences. As you proceed, keep in mind that healing is about creating a meaningful and hopeful future by learning to live with your loss as well as your hope. Although grief will undoubtedly be a part of your journey, there is also hope for recovery, development, and rejuvenation. Your hopes and dreams are like paint waiting to be applied to the canvas of the future, which is to honor the love and loss that have led you to this moment.

CONCLUSION

This book explores the journey of empathy, comprehension, and hope in recovering from miscarriage and stillbirth. We took this route in order to recognize the severe loss and suffering that far too many people and families go through, frequently in silence. Our intention was to offer a source of comfort, direction, and resilience while illuminating the psychological and physical intricacies of these experiences.

We have looked at the many facets of grief in these pages, covering everything from the first shock and sadness to the protracted process of healing and acceptance. We have discussed the value of getting support from friends, family, and professionals as well as the efficacy of self-care and self-compassion.

We have witnessed the tremendous strength of the human spirit and the ability to grow even in the face of severe loss by hearing the stories of those who have traveled this difficult path. We now understand the value of rituals and celebrations, the power of accepting and processing grief, and the necessity of paying tribute to the children who departed from us too soon.

This book has also given readers a foundation for understanding the physiological and medical aspects of miscarriage, providing details on possible causes, safeguards, and remedies. We now possess more knowledge, which promotes candid discussions and well-informed choices.

Above all, the message of hope is at the heart of this book. We've learned that healing isn't a straight line; it's a very personal journey. While the pain of loss will never go away, it can be transformed into a source of strength and resilience.

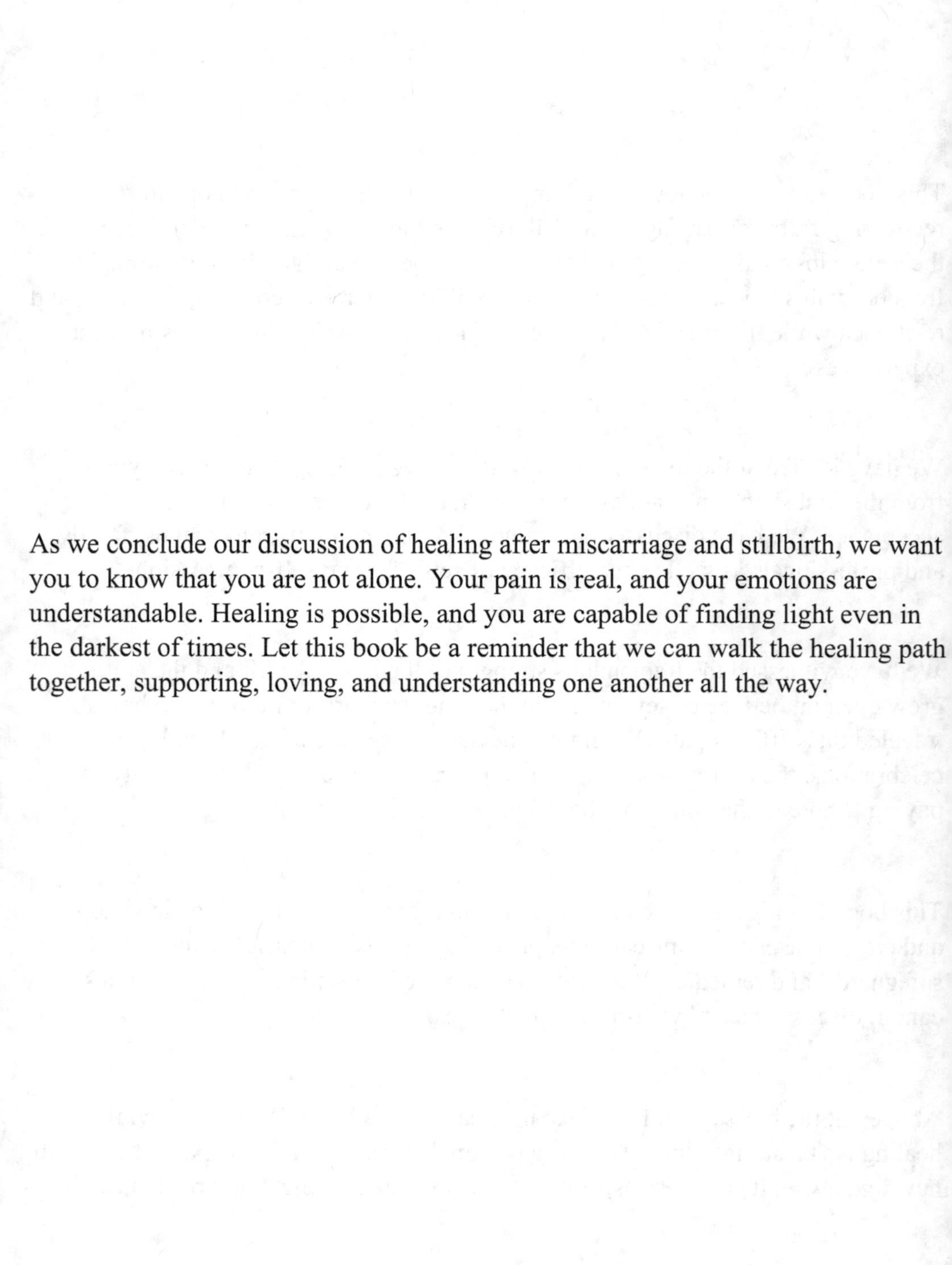

As we conclude our discussion of healing after miscarriage and stillbirth, we want you to know that you are not alone. Your pain is real, and your emotions are understandable. Healing is possible, and you are capable of finding light even in the darkest of times. Let this book be a reminder that we can walk the healing path together, supporting, loving, and understanding one another all the way.